OPTIMAL GUT HEALTH

A Physician's Guide to Relieving Constipation Through Fiber Therapy

By

Calvin M. Duncan

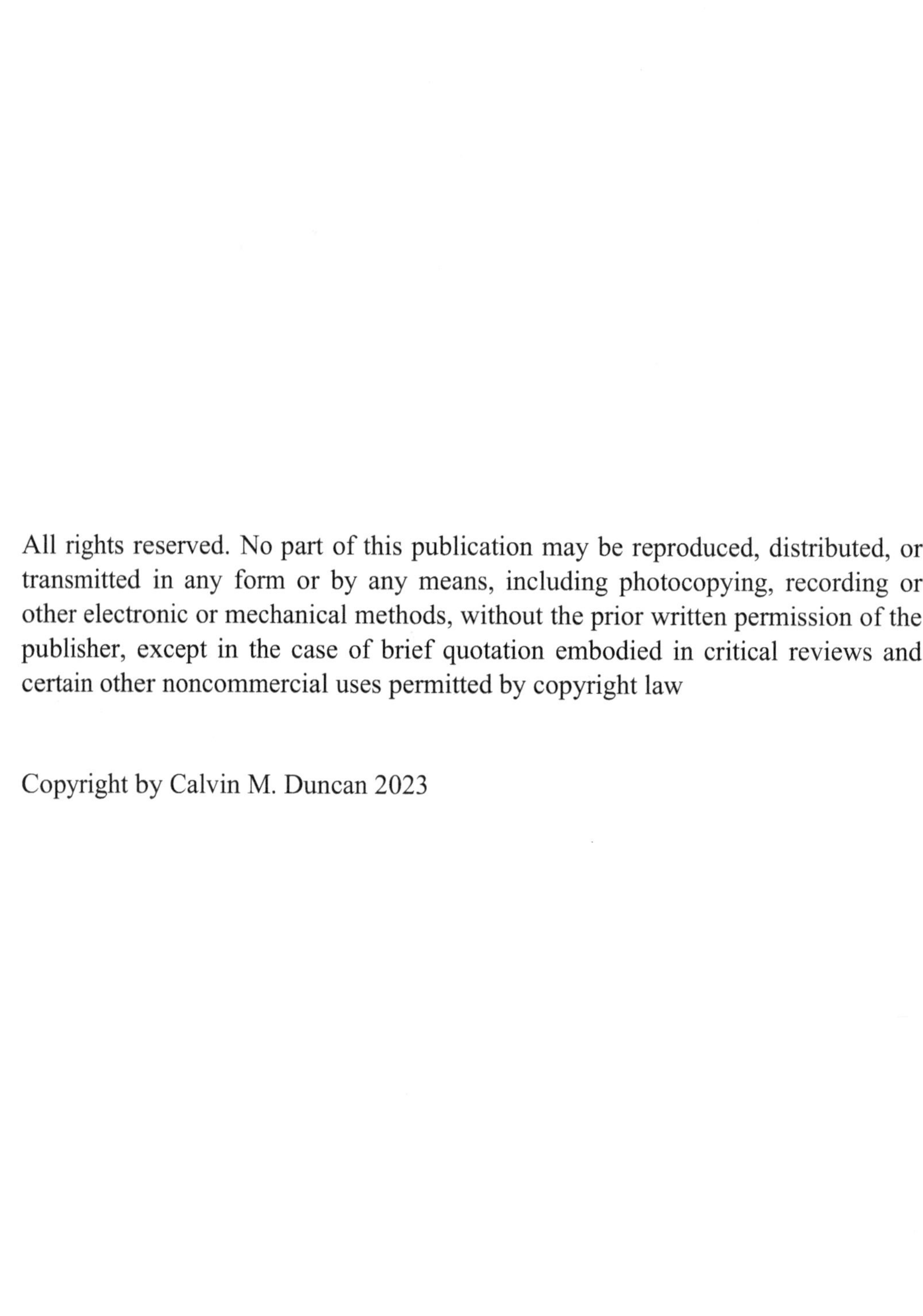

Table of Contents

CHAPTER ONE

Understanding Constipation: Unraveling the Causes

Constipation, a prevalent gastrointestinal woe, affects individuals across diverse demographics. Characterized by infrequent bowel movements, difficulty in passing stools, and a pervasive sense of incomplete evacuation, constipation can significantly impede one's daily life. While occasional constipation is considered normal, chronic cases warrant a comprehensive exploration of the multifaceted causes that contribute to its onset.

A pivotal factor in the genesis of constipation lies in dietary choices. The absence of an adequate intake of dietary fiber can disrupt the delicate balance of the digestive system. Fiber, essential for adding bulk to stool, facilitates its smooth passage through the intestinal tract. When the diet lacks fiber, transit time in the intestines elongates, resulting in hardened stools that are challenging to expel. Dehydration compounds the issue, as water is indispensable for maintaining optimal bowel function. Inadequate fluid intake can lead to dry and compacted stools, exacerbating constipation.

Physical activity, or the lack thereof, plays a pivotal role in bowel regularity. A sedentary lifestyle, characterized by minimal physical movement, can induce sluggish bowel function. Regular exercise serves to stimulate the muscles of the intestines, promoting the smooth transit of stool. The absence of physical activity, conversely, contributes to a slowdown in the digestive process, culminating in constipation.

Certain medications, often prescribed for various health conditions, can inadvertently lead to constipation. Opioid pain medications, antacids containing aluminum or calcium, certain antidepressants, and antispasmodic drugs are recognized culprits. These medications interfere with the rhythmic contractions of the intestines, impeding bowel movements. Individuals on such medications must be cognizant of this potential side effect and collaborate with healthcare providers to implement preventive measures.

Neurological disorders, such as Parkinson's disease and multiple sclerosis, introduce a complex dimension to the constipation narrative. These conditions affect the nerves controlling bowel function, disrupting the coordinated muscle contractions essential for regular bowel movements. Understanding the intricate interplay between neurological health and gastrointestinal function is vital for effective constipation management in individuals grappling with these disorders.

Hormonal imbalances, a facet often overlooked, can significantly impact bowel habits. Fluctuations in estrogen and progesterone levels, particularly during pregnancy and menstruation, can induce constipation. The pressure exerted by a growing uterus during pregnancy, coupled with

hormonal changes, contributes to constipation in expectant mothers. Acknowledging the role of hormones in gastrointestinal health is imperative for a nuanced understanding of constipation triggers.

Structural issues within the gastrointestinal tract, such as bowel obstructions or blockages, can manifest as constipation. Conditions like colorectal cancer, intestinal strictures, or impacted feces can impede the smooth flow of stool. Identifying and addressing these structural abnormalities is pivotal in managing constipation and averting potential complications.

Irritable Bowel Syndrome (IBS), a prevalent gastrointestinal disorder, further underscores the complexity of constipation's etiology. IBS, with its constipation-predominant subtype (IBS-C), presents with abdominal pain, bloating, and altered bowel habits. While the precise cause of IBS remains elusive, aberrations in gut motility, visceral hypersensitivity, and abnormal gut-brain interactions collectively contribute to its manifestation.

Advancing age brings with it a natural decline in muscle tone, impacting the muscles of the digestive tract. This age-related muscle weakness results in slower bowel movements, a phenomenon compounded by diminishing nerve responsiveness in the intestines. Recognizing the influence of aging on gastrointestinal function is essential for tailoring interventions that address constipation in the elderly effectively.

Psychological factors, particularly stress and anxiety, cast a long shadow on digestive health. The intricate gut-brain axis, a bidirectional communication system, regulates bowel function. Stress-induced alterations in gut motility and sensitivity can lead to constipation. Holistic constipation management necessitates the integration of relaxation techniques and stress management into the treatment paradigm.

Certain systemic diseases, such as hypothyroidism and diabetes, exert a profound influence on bowel function. Hypothyroidism, characterized by an underactive thyroid gland, slows down metabolism and impacts intestinal muscle function. Diabetes, especially when poorly controlled, can damage nerves in the intestines, contributing to constipation. Effectively managing these underlying systemic conditions is imperative for addressing constipation at its roots.

In conclusion, constipation emerges as a nuanced and intricate condition with a multitude of causative factors. Understanding the complex interplay between dietary choices, lifestyle, medications, neurological health, hormonal balance, structural issues, and systemic diseases is critical for formulating a comprehensive approach to constipation management. A holistic strategy, encompassing dietary modifications, lifestyle adjustments, and, when necessary, medical interventions, is indispensable for restoring optimal bowel function and overall gastrointestinal health. By unraveling the intricate tapestry of causes, healthcare professionals and individuals alike can collaboratively navigate the path towards alleviating the burden of constipation and fostering enduring digestive well-being.

CHAPTER TWO

The Role of Fiber in Digestive Health

Digestive health is a cornerstone of overall well-being, influencing various aspects of our daily lives. Within the realm of digestive health, the role of dietary fiber emerges as a crucial factor in maintaining optimal functioning. Fiber, a component predominantly found in plant-based foods, plays a multifaceted role in supporting digestive processes, from promoting regular bowel movements to contributing to a healthy gut microbiome. In this comprehensive exploration, we delve into the various facets of fiber and its impact on digestive health, considering its sources, types, recommended intake, and the potential benefits it offers.

Fiber, often referred to as roughage or bulk, is a type of carbohydrate that the body cannot digest or absorb. Unlike other carbohydrates, such as sugars and starches, fiber passes through the digestive system relatively intact. It is primarily derived from plant-based foods, including fruits, vegetables, whole grains, legumes, nuts, and seeds. Fiber is classified into two main types: soluble and insoluble.

Soluble fiber dissolves in water to form a gel-like substance, which can help lower blood cholesterol and stabilize blood sugar levels. Good sources of soluble fiber include oats, barley, beans, lentils, fruits, and vegetables. On the other hand, insoluble fiber adds bulk to the stool and aids in moving it through the digestive tract. Whole wheat, nuts, seeds, and the skins of fruits and vegetables are rich in insoluble fiber.

As part of the digestive process, fiber undergoes a unique journey through the gastrointestinal tract. Upon ingestion, fiber-rich foods enter the stomach, where they are broken down into smaller particles. Unlike other nutrients, fiber resists digestion in the stomach and small intestine. Instead, it moves largely undigested into the colon, or large intestine.

In the colon, bacteria ferment some types of fiber, producing short-chain fatty acids (SCFAs) as byproducts. These SCFAs serve as a source of energy for the cells lining the colon and play a role in maintaining gut health. The fermentation process also contributes to the production of gases, which can influence bowel regularity and overall digestive function.

One of the most well-known benefits of fiber in digestive health is its role in promoting regular bowel movements. Insoluble fiber, in particular, adds bulk to the stool, making it softer and easier to pass through the intestines. This prevents constipation and facilitates the smooth movement of waste through the digestive tract.

Soluble fiber, by forming a gel-like substance in the digestive tract, can also contribute to bowel regularity. It helps regulate the consistency of stool and, in some cases, may be beneficial in managing diarrhea by absorbing excess water.

Constipation, a common digestive complaint, is often linked to insufficient fiber intake. A diet lacking in fiber can result in slow transit time through the intestines, leading to hard and difficult-to-pass stools. Increasing fiber intake, along with adequate hydration, is a foundational strategy in managing and preventing constipation.

For individuals prone to constipation, incorporating a variety of fiber-rich foods into their diet can make a substantial difference. Whole grains, fruits, vegetables, and legumes provide a spectrum of fibers that contribute to overall digestive health. Additionally, fiber supplements, such as psyllium husk or methylcellulose, may be recommended under the guidance of healthcare professionals to address constipation.

Fiber plays a crucial role in weight management and promoting a feeling of fullness or satiety. High-fiber foods generally require more chewing, which can slow down the eating process and provide the brain with signals of fullness. This can contribute to better portion control and, consequently, weight maintenance or weight loss.

Moreover, certain types of soluble fiber, such as beta-glucans found in oats, have been associated with improved metabolic health. These fibers may help regulate blood sugar levels and reduce the risk of developing insulin resistance, a factor linked to obesity and type 2 diabetes.

Dietary fiber, particularly soluble fiber, plays a pivotal role in regulating blood sugar levels. When consumed with carbohydrates, fiber can slow down the absorption of sugars, preventing rapid spikes in blood glucose. This is particularly beneficial for individuals with diabetes or those at risk of developing the condition.

Incorporating high-fiber foods into meals can contribute to better glycemic control, reducing the post-meal rise in blood sugar. The viscous nature of soluble fiber also aids in trapping sugars, allowing for a more gradual release into the bloodstream.

Fiber has a positive impact on cardiovascular health, primarily through its role in managing cholesterol levels. Soluble fiber binds to cholesterol molecules in the digestive tract, preventing their absorption into the bloodstream. This, in turn, leads to a reduction in blood cholesterol levels, specifically low-density lipoprotein (LDL) cholesterol, often referred to as "bad" cholesterol.

Oats, barley, beans, and fruits such as apples and citrus fruits are renowned for their cholesterol-lowering effects. Including these foods in a heart-healthy diet can contribute to the prevention of cardiovascular diseases.

The gut microbiome, a complex ecosystem of trillions of microorganisms residing in the digestive tract, plays a pivotal role in digestive and overall health. Fiber serves as a prebiotic, a substance that nourishes beneficial bacteria in the colon. These bacteria ferment fiber, producing metabolites, including SCFAs, which contribute to a healthy gut environment.

A diverse and thriving gut microbiome is associated with enhanced immune function, reduced inflammation, and protection against various gastrointestinal disorders. Fiber-rich foods, therefore, contribute not only to digestive health but also to the broader aspects of immune function and overall well-being.

Adequate fiber intake has been linked to a reduced risk of colorectal cancer. Insoluble fiber, in particular, adds bulk to the stool, which speeds up its transit through the colon. This, in turn, minimizes the time that potentially harmful substances in the stool are in contact with the intestinal lining.

Furthermore, the fermentation of soluble fiber in the colon produces SCFAs, which have been associated with anti-cancer properties. These SCFAs may help regulate cell growth and apoptosis, contributing to the prevention of colorectal cancer.

To harness the full spectrum of benefits that fiber offers, it's essential to understand the different types of fiber and their dietary sources. As mentioned earlier, soluble fiber is found in foods like oats, barley, beans, lentils, fruits, and vegetables. Insoluble fiber is abundant in whole wheat, nuts, seeds, and the skins of fruits and vegetables.

The recommended daily intake of fiber varies by age, sex, and life stage. In general, adults are advised to consume between 25 to 38 grams of fiber per day, depending on factors such as age and gender. However, population-based studies consistently indicate that many individuals fall short of meeting these recommendations.

Despite the recognized benefits of fiber, there are challenges associated with increasing fiber intake. Some individuals may experience bloating, gas, or abdominal discomfort when significantly changing their fiber intake. Gradual adjustments, along with increased water consumption, can help mitigate these symptoms.

It's also crucial to note that not all sources of fiber are created equal. Highly processed foods may contain added fibers that do not provide the same health benefits as naturally occurring fibers in whole foods. Therefore, a focus on a diverse and whole-food-based diet remains essential for reaping the full spectrum of fiber-related advantages.

In conclusion, the role of fiber in digestive health is profound and multifaceted. From promoting regular bowel movements to influencing weight management, blood sugar regulation, cardiovascular health, and the prevention of colorectal cancer, fiber stands as a foundational element in the pursuit of overall well-being.

Understanding the diverse types of fiber, their dietary sources, and the recommended intake is key to harnessing the benefits effectively. A balanced and varied diet that incorporates a rich array of fiber from fruits, vegetables, whole grains, legumes, nuts, and seeds is fundamental for digestive health and beyond.

As the nexus between nutrition and health continues to be unraveled, the significance of fiber in fostering a resilient and thriving digestive system cannot be overstated. Embracing dietary habits that prioritize fiber-rich foods contributes not only to the optimization of digestive function but also to the broader canvas of long-term health and vitality. In this journey towards well-being, fiber emerges as a stalwart ally, navigating the intricate pathways of the digestive system and fortifying the foundations of holistic health.

CHAPTER THREE

Fiber Types and Their Impact on Constipation

Constipation, a prevalent digestive issue affecting people worldwide, often finds its solution in the incorporation of fiber into one's diet. Fiber, the indigestible part of plant-based foods, plays a pivotal role in promoting bowel regularity and preventing constipation. However, not all fibers are created equal. Understanding the different types of fiber and their distinct impacts on digestive health is crucial for effectively addressing and preventing constipation.

Soluble Fiber: The Gel-Forming Hero

Soluble fiber, as the name implies, dissolves in water to form a gel-like substance. This unique property makes soluble fiber particularly effective in managing constipation. Foods rich in soluble fiber include oats, beans, lentils, fruits, and vegetables. When soluble fiber comes into contact with water, it transforms into a viscous gel that slows down the digestive process.

The gel-forming nature of soluble fiber serves multiple purposes in the context of constipation. Firstly, it helps soften the stool by absorbing water, making it easier to pass through the digestive tract. This is especially beneficial for individuals experiencing hard, dry stools that contribute to constipation.

Secondly, the gel created by soluble fiber adds bulk to the stool. This increased bulk stimulates the muscles in the intestines, promoting the rhythmic contractions necessary for effective bowel movements. As the stool moves through the colon, the presence of soluble fiber facilitates its smooth passage.

Insoluble Fiber: Nature's Broom

While soluble fiber forms a gel, insoluble fiber remains relatively unchanged as it passes through the digestive tract. Insoluble fiber is found in foods like whole grains, nuts, seeds, and the skin of fruits and vegetables. Often referred to as "roughage" or "nature's broom," insoluble fiber adds bulk to the stool and accelerates its transit through the intestines.

The primary role of insoluble fiber is to promote regular bowel movements by preventing constipation. As it moves through the digestive tract, insoluble fiber helps prevent the stool from becoming too hard and aids in its timely elimination. By providing mechanical support and promoting the movement of stool, insoluble fiber contributes to overall digestive health.

Resistant Starch: Fuel for Gut Bacteria

Resistant starch is a type of carbohydrate that resists digestion in the small intestine and reaches the colon intact. While not classified as traditional dietary fiber, resistant starch exhibits similar properties in terms of its impact on digestive health. Foods high in resistant starch include green bananas, legumes, and certain whole grains.

Once in the colon, resistant starch becomes a source of fuel for beneficial gut bacteria. The fermentation of resistant starch produces short-chain fatty acids, which play a crucial role in maintaining gut health. These fatty acids not only nourish the cells lining the colon but also contribute to the regulation of bowel movements.

Prebiotic Fiber: Nurturing Gut Microbiota

Prebiotic fiber refers to a type of fiber that serves as a nutrient source for beneficial bacteria in the gut. While soluble and insoluble fibers can have prebiotic effects, certain fibers are specifically recognized for their ability to support the growth and activity of probiotics. Foods rich in prebiotic fibers include garlic, onions, leeks, and certain fruits and vegetables.

A healthy balance of gut microbiota is essential for optimal digestive function. Prebiotic fibers promote the proliferation of beneficial bacteria, which, in turn, contribute to the breakdown of complex carbohydrates, the production of essential nutrients, and the regulation of immune function. A flourishing gut microbiome is closely linked to overall gut health, including the prevention of constipation.

Fiber-Rich Foods: Building a Constipation-Resistant Diet

Achieving the optimal balance of fiber types involves incorporating a variety of fiber-rich foods into one's diet. A diverse and colorful array of fruits, vegetables, whole grains, legumes, nuts, and seeds ensures a broad spectrum of both soluble and insoluble fibers.

Fruits such as apples, pears, and berries are excellent sources of soluble fiber, contributing to the formation of the gel that aids in softening the stool. Additionally, the skin of fruits provides insoluble fiber, enhancing bulk and promoting efficient bowel movements.

Vegetables, particularly leafy greens, carrots, and broccoli, offer a combination of soluble and insoluble fibers. Including a variety of vegetables in daily meals provides essential nutrients and supports digestive health.

Whole grains, including oats, brown rice, and quinoa, provide a hearty dose of both soluble and insoluble fibers. These grains contribute to the overall fiber content of the diet, supporting digestive regularity.

Legumes, such as beans and lentils, are rich in soluble fiber, offering both a protein boost and digestive benefits. Including legumes in meals adds bulk to the stool and supports healthy bowel movements.

Nuts and seeds, including almonds, chia seeds, and flaxseeds, provide a mix of soluble and insoluble fibers. These nutrient-dense foods contribute not only to digestive health but also to overall well-being.

Fiber Supplements: Bridging the Gap

While a balanced and fiber-rich diet is the ideal way to obtain the necessary nutrients, fiber supplements can be a convenient option for those struggling to meet their fiber needs through food alone. Fiber supplements come in various forms, including powders, capsules, and chewable tablets, and they often contain isolated forms of soluble or insoluble fiber.

Psyllium husk is a common ingredient in many fiber supplements and is particularly rich in soluble fiber. It has been shown to be effective in softening the stool and promoting regular bowel movements. Other supplemental fibers, such as methylcellulose and wheat dextrin, also contribute to increased fiber intake and can be useful for individuals seeking additional support.

However, it's crucial to approach fiber supplementation with caution and under the guidance of a healthcare professional. Sudden and excessive increases in fiber intake, whether through diet or supplements, can lead to bloating, gas, and abdominal discomfort. Gradual adjustments and adequate hydration are essential when incorporating fiber supplements into one's routine.

Impact on Constipation: The Mechanisms at Play

Understanding how different types of fiber impact constipation involves examining the mechanisms through which they exert their beneficial effects. Soluble fiber, with its gel-forming nature, softens the stool and adds bulk, facilitating its smooth passage through the intestines. This is particularly helpful for individuals experiencing constipation characterized by hard and dry stools.

Insoluble fiber, acting as nature's broom, contributes to the mechanical aspects of digestion. By adding bulk to the stool and promoting its movement through the colon, insoluble fiber prevents constipation by ensuring timely elimination. This is especially beneficial for those prone to irregular bowel movements or difficulty passing stool.

The fermentation of resistant starch in the colon produces short-chain fatty acids, contributing to the overall health of the gut. While not a direct cure for constipation, the supportive role of resistant starch in maintaining gut microbiota may indirectly influence bowel regularity by promoting a healthy and balanced digestive environment.

Prebiotic fibers, by nourishing beneficial gut bacteria, contribute to the intricate ecosystem of the gut microbiome. A thriving gut microbiota is associated with various health benefits, including improved digestion and immune function. While not a direct remedy for constipation, a healthy gut microbiome sets the stage for optimal digestive health.

Tailoring Fiber Intake to Individual Needs

The impact of fiber on constipation is not a one-size-fits-all scenario. Individual responses to different types and amounts of fiber can vary based on factors such as age, sex, overall health, and underlying medical conditions. Tailoring fiber intake to individual needs requires a nuanced approach, taking into account various factors that may influence digestive health.

For some individuals, increasing soluble fiber may be particularly beneficial, especially if constipation is associated with hard and dry stools. Soluble fiber's ability to form a gel and soften the stool addresses this specific issue, making bowel movements more comfortable.

Others may benefit from a focus on insoluble fiber if their constipation is related to a lack of bulk in the stool or sluggish intestinal transit. Insoluble fiber adds volume to the stool and promotes its movement through the colon, addressing these specific concerns.

In cases where gut microbiota health is a priority, emphasizing prebiotic fibers and foods rich in resistant starch may be beneficial. These fibers provide essential nutrients for beneficial bacteria, contributing to a balanced and flourishing gut microbiome.

The Importance of Adequate Hydration

While fiber is a key player in preventing constipation, its effectiveness is closely tied to hydration. Water plays a crucial role in the digestion of fiber, especially soluble fiber, which absorbs water to form a gel. Without adequate hydration, the benefits of fiber may be compromised, and constipation could persist.

It's recommended to drink plenty of water throughout the day, especially when increasing fiber intake. Hydration not only ensures the proper functioning of fiber but also supports overall digestive health. Individuals prone to constipation should be mindful of their water intake and aim to maintain a healthy balance.

Challenges and Considerations

While fiber is generally celebrated for its positive impact on digestive health, there are challenges and considerations to keep in mind. Rapidly increasing fiber intake, whether through diet or supplements, can lead to bloating, gas, and abdominal discomfort. This is particularly true for individuals who are not accustomed to a high-fiber diet.

To mitigate these challenges, it's advisable to gradually introduce fiber into the diet and monitor individual responses. Additionally, considering the diverse sources of fiber and incorporating a variety of foods can help prevent discomfort associated with specific types of fiber.

Individuals with certain medical conditions, such as irritable bowel syndrome (IBS) or inflammatory bowel disease (IBD), may need to approach fiber intake with caution. In some cases, specific types of fiber or certain foods may exacerbate symptoms, and personalized guidance from a healthcare professional is essential.

Conclusion

In the intricate web of digestive health, fiber emerges as a fundamental player in the prevention and management of constipation. The distinct impacts of soluble fiber, insoluble fiber, resistant starch, and prebiotic fiber contribute to a comprehensive approach to digestive well-being.

By incorporating a diverse range of fiber-rich foods into the diet, individuals can support the intricate mechanisms of the digestive system. Whether through fruits, vegetables, whole grains, legumes, nuts, or seeds, each food source brings its unique blend of soluble and insoluble fibers, contributing to optimal bowel regularity.

Understanding that the impact of fiber on constipation is multifaceted allows for a tailored approach to individual needs. Whether seeking to soften hard stools, add bulk to the stool, or nurture a healthy gut microbiome, the diverse array of fiber types provides a range of solutions.

As individuals embark on the journey of optimizing their fiber intake, it's crucial to approach the process with mindfulness and consideration. Gradual adjustments, adequate hydration, and attention to individual responses can help navigate potential challenges associated with increased fiber consumption.

In the realm of digestive health, fiber stands as a versatile ally, offering not only relief from constipation but also contributing to overall well-being. By understanding the nuances of fiber types and their impact on constipation, individuals can empower themselves to make informed dietary choices that support a healthy and harmonious digestive system.

CHAPTER FOUR

Crafting Your Fiber-Rich Diet Plan

A well-balanced and nutrient-rich diet is the cornerstone of good health, and when it comes to promoting digestive wellness, the inclusion of an adequate amount of dietary fiber is paramount. Crafting a fiber-rich diet plan involves thoughtful consideration of food choices, meal composition, and lifestyle factors to ensure optimal bowel regularity and prevent constipation. In this exploration, we delve into the art and science of designing a personalized and sustainable fiber-rich diet that fosters digestive health.

The Art of Food Selection

Fruits: Nature's Sweet Fiber Bounty

Fruits are not only a delicious addition to any diet but also a rich source of dietary fiber. Incorporating a variety of fruits into your daily meals ensures a diverse range of fiber types, including soluble and insoluble fibers. Berries, such as strawberries, blueberries, and raspberries, are not only packed with antioxidants but also high in soluble fiber, contributing to the softening of stool.

Apples, with their skin intact, provide a good dose of soluble fiber, specifically pectin, which forms a gel-like substance in the digestive tract. Pears, plums, and kiwi are additional fruit options that contribute both soluble and insoluble fibers to support overall digestive health.

Vegetables: A Colorful Fiber Palette

Vegetables are a nutritional powerhouse, offering an array of vitamins, minerals, and, importantly, dietary fiber. Leafy greens like spinach, kale, and Swiss chard are not only rich in nutrients but also provide both soluble and insoluble fibers. Cruciferous vegetables, including broccoli, cauliflower, and Brussels sprouts, add bulk to the stool and contribute to efficient bowel movements.

Carrots, sweet potatoes, and bell peppers are excellent sources of soluble fiber, supporting the gel-forming properties that aid in softening the stool. Including a variety of colorful vegetables in your diet not only ensures a diverse nutrient profile but also provides a spectrum of fiber types for comprehensive digestive support.

Whole Grains: The Fiber Foundation

Whole grains form the foundation of a fiber-rich diet, offering a robust mix of soluble and insoluble fibers. Brown rice, quinoa, oats, barley, and whole wheat are examples of whole grains that

contribute to the overall fiber content of meals. Choosing whole grains over refined grains ensures the retention of the bran and germ, where the majority of the fiber is found.

Whole grain bread, pasta, and cereals provide convenient options for incorporating fiber into your diet. When selecting these products, it's essential to check labels for whole grain content and opt for those with minimal processing. The fiber content in whole grains contributes to the bulk and softness of the stool, promoting regular bowel movements.

Legumes: Fiber and Protein Powerhouse

Legumes, including beans, lentils, and chickpeas, are not only rich in protein but also a significant source of dietary fiber. Both soluble and insoluble fibers are present in legumes, making them a versatile addition to various dishes. Black beans, kidney beans, and navy beans, among others, can be included in salads, soups, or as a side dish to boost fiber intake.

Lentils, known for their high fiber content, cook quickly and can be incorporated into a variety of recipes. Hummus, made from chickpeas, provides a flavorful and fiber-rich dip or spread. Including legumes in your diet adds both soluble and insoluble fibers, contributing to digestive health and overall well-being.

Nuts and Seeds: Nutrient-Dense Fiber Boosters

Nuts and seeds are not only packed with essential nutrients like omega-3 fatty acids and antioxidants but also contribute to the fiber content of your diet. Almonds, chia seeds, flaxseeds, and walnuts are excellent choices for a fiber-rich snack or topping for yogurt and salads.

While nuts and seeds contain more soluble fiber, they also provide insoluble fiber, adding bulk to the stool. Including a variety of nuts and seeds in your diet not only enhances flavor and texture but also contributes to the overall fiber composition of your meals.

Dairy and Alternatives: A Balanced Approach

Dairy products and their alternatives can be part of a fiber-rich diet, although they are not typically high in fiber. Choosing low-fat or fat-free dairy options helps strike a balance between nutrient intake and overall dietary goals. Yogurt, especially if it contains probiotics, contributes to gut health, while also providing a small amount of dietary fiber.

Plant-based alternatives, such as almond milk or soy milk, may be fortified with fiber, offering additional options for those with dietary preferences or restrictions. While not a primary source of fiber, incorporating dairy and alternatives mindfully ensures a well-rounded and diverse nutrient intake.

The Science of Meal Composition

Breakfast: Fiber-Packed Start

Crafting a fiber-rich diet plan begins with a nutrient-dense breakfast that sets the tone for the day. Starting the morning with whole grain cereal, oats, or a fiber-enriched smoothie provides an early boost of both soluble and insoluble fibers. Adding fruits, nuts, or seeds to your breakfast further enhances the fiber content while contributing essential vitamins and minerals.

Whole grain toast with avocado or nut butter is another nutritious breakfast option. Including a variety of foods ensures a mix of fiber types, supporting digestion and promoting sustained energy throughout the morning.

Lunch: Veggie-Packed Plates

Lunchtime offers ample opportunities to incorporate fiber-rich foods into your meals. Opting for a colorful salad with a mix of leafy greens, vegetables, and a variety of proteins such as grilled chicken, tofu, or legumes ensures a balanced and fiber-packed plate. Adding quinoa or brown rice as a base enhances the fiber content while providing additional nutrients.

Whole grain wraps or sandwiches with lean protein, fresh vegetables, and a spread of hummus or avocado offer a portable and satisfying lunch option. Including a side of raw vegetables or a piece of fruit further boosts fiber intake, contributing to overall digestive health.

Snacks: Smart and Fiber-Focused

Snacking can be an opportunity to sneak in additional fiber between meals. Opting for whole fruits, raw vegetables with hummus, or a handful of nuts and seeds provides a nutrient-dense and fiber-rich snack. Greek yogurt with added berries or a sprinkle of granola is another satisfying option that contributes both protein and fiber.

When selecting packaged snacks, it's essential to read labels and choose those with minimal processing and added sugars. Whole food snacks that include a combination of fiber types help maintain energy levels and support digestive wellness.

Dinner: Balanced and Varied

Dinner is an excellent time to create a well-balanced and fiber-rich meal. Including a variety of vegetables as a side dish or incorporating them into main courses ensures a diverse range of fiber types. Stir-fries with colorful vegetables, lean protein, and a serving of brown rice or quinoa offer a balanced and satisfying dinner option.

Vegetarian or bean-based dishes, such as lentil stew or chickpea curry, provide both protein and fiber. Whole grain pasta or noodles with tomato-based sauces and a medley of vegetables contribute to a hearty and fiber-focused dinner.

Lifestyle Considerations

Hydration: The Companion to Fiber

Adequate hydration is a crucial companion to a fiber-rich diet. Water plays a pivotal role in the effectiveness of soluble fiber, enabling it to form the necessary gel-like substance that softens the stool. Without proper hydration, the benefits of fiber may be diminished, and constipation could persist.

It's recommended to drink plenty of water throughout the day, especially when increasing fiber intake. Herbal teas and infused water with fruits or herbs can add variety to hydration while contributing to overall fluid balance.

Physical Activity: Stimulating Digestive Health

Regular physical activity complements a fiber-rich diet in promoting optimal digestive health. Exercise stimulates the muscles in the intestines, supporting the natural rhythm of bowel movements. Incorporating both aerobic exercises, such as walking or jogging, and strength training exercises into your routine contributes to overall well-being.

Aim for at least 150 minutes of moderate-intensity exercise per week, as recommended by health guidelines. Finding activities you enjoy not only supports digestive health but also enhances your overall fitness and vitality.

Mindful Eating: Enhancing Digestive Awareness

Practicing mindful eating involves paying attention to the sensory experience of eating, being present during meals, and listening to your body's hunger and fullness cues. Chewing food thoroughly and savoring the flavors enhances the digestive process and supports nutrient absorption.

Mindful eating also involves recognizing the signals of satiety and avoiding overeating. This approach to eating fosters a positive relationship with food and contributes to overall digestive wellness.

Gradual Adjustments: Allowing for Adaptation

When transitioning to a fiber-rich diet, it's advisable to make gradual adjustments to allow your digestive system to adapt. Rapidly increasing fiber intake can lead to bloating, gas, and abdominal discomfort. Start by incorporating one or two fiber-rich foods at a time and gradually increasing the variety and quantity.

Fiber supplements can be a convenient option for those struggling to meet their fiber needs through food alone. However, it's crucial to approach supplementation with caution and under the guidance of a healthcare professional. Sudden and excessive increases in fiber intake, whether through diet or supplements, can lead to digestive discomfort.

Addressing Challenges and Individual Needs

Food Sensitivities and Intolerances

Individuals with specific food sensitivities or intolerances may need to tailor their fiber-rich diet plan accordingly. For those with lactose intolerance or sensitivity to gluten, alternative options such as lactose-free dairy or gluten-free whole grains can be considered.

It's essential to listen to your body and be mindful of any adverse reactions to certain foods. Working with a healthcare professional or a registered dietitian can provide personalized guidance based on individual dietary needs and restrictions.

Gastrointestinal Conditions

Certain gastrointestinal conditions, such as irritable bowel syndrome (IBS) or inflammatory bowel disease (IBD), may require a more individualized approach to a fiber-rich diet. Some individuals with IBS may find relief with a low-FODMAP diet, which temporarily restricts certain fermentable carbohydrates that can contribute to symptoms.

In cases of IBD, where inflammation in the digestive tract is present, dietary adjustments may be needed based on individual tolerances. It's crucial for individuals with gastrointestinal conditions to work closely with healthcare professionals to create a dietary plan that supports digestive health while managing specific symptoms.

Medications and Interactions

Certain medications may interact with dietary fiber or impact its absorption. Individuals taking medications should be aware of potential interactions and consult with their healthcare provider for guidance. For example, some medications may need to be taken separately from fiber supplements to optimize absorption.

It's advisable to inform healthcare providers about any dietary supplements or significant changes to your diet to ensure a comprehensive understanding of your overall health and potential interactions.

Monitoring and Adjusting

Crafting a fiber-rich diet plan is not a one-time event but an ongoing process that requires monitoring and adjustments. Paying attention to how your body responds to different foods, meal compositions, and lifestyle factors allows for informed decision-making. Keep a food journal or diary to track your dietary choices, digestive symptoms, and overall well-being.

If you experience persistent digestive issues or changes in bowel habits, it's essential to seek guidance from a healthcare professional. Chronic constipation or other digestive concerns may warrant further investigation to identify underlying causes and develop an appropriate treatment plan.

Conclusion

Crafting a fiber-rich diet plan is a personalized journey that involves both the art and science of food selection and meal composition. By incorporating a variety of fiber-rich foods, such as fruits, vegetables, whole grains, legumes, nuts, and seeds, individuals can create a diverse and nutrient-dense diet that supports optimal digestive health.

The science of meal composition involves thoughtful consideration of nutrient balance, fiber types, and overall dietary goals. Designing well-rounded and satisfying meals for breakfast, lunch, and dinner ensures a consistent intake of fiber throughout the day. Snacks and hydration contribute to maintaining energy levels and supporting digestive wellness.

Lifestyle considerations, including hydration, physical activity, mindful eating, and gradual adjustments, play a crucial role in enhancing the effectiveness of a fiber-rich diet. Addressing challenges and individual needs, such as food sensitivities, gastrointestinal conditions, and medication interactions, requires a tailored approach and collaboration with healthcare professionals.

Monitoring and adjusting your dietary plan based on individual responses and overall well-being is an integral part of the process. A fiber-rich diet is not a rigid prescription but a flexible and sustainable approach to promoting digestive health. By embracing the art and science of crafting a fiber-rich diet plan, individuals can take proactive steps towards achieving and maintaining optimal digestive wellness.

CHAPTER FIVE

The Power of Hydration: Supporting Bowel Regularity

Water – a simple, transparent liquid that constitutes the very essence of life. It is the elixir that sustains every living organism on Earth, and its significance extends far beyond quenching our thirst. Among its many vital roles, hydration plays a pivotal role in maintaining bowel regularity, a fundamental aspect of digestive health that often goes unnoticed in our daily lives.

Water: The Essence of Life

Before delving into the intricate relationship between hydration and bowel regularity, it is essential to underscore the unparalleled importance of water in sustaining life. The human body, on average, is composed of about 60% water, highlighting its integral role in various physiological processes. From facilitating nutrient transport to regulating body temperature and supporting cellular functions, water is the silent conductor of the symphony of life.

The Digestive Symphony: Hydration's Role

Within the symphony of bodily functions, the digestive system is a complex orchestra of processes that transform the food we consume into essential nutrients. Hydration emerges as a key conductor in this digestive symphony, influencing the entire gastrointestinal tract's performance.

As food travels through the digestive system, it encounters different environments, each requiring optimal hydration for efficient functioning. In the mouth, saliva, a watery secretion, initiates the process of digestion by breaking down carbohydrates. As food progresses through the stomach and small intestine, digestive juices and enzymes, suspended in a water-based medium, continue the breakdown of nutrients.

The importance of hydration becomes particularly evident in the large intestine, the final segment of the digestive tract. Here, water plays a crucial role in shaping the consistency of stool and facilitating its smooth passage. Adequate hydration ensures that the digestive process unfolds seamlessly, promoting the absorption of nutrients and the elimination of waste.

Hydration and Bowel Regularity

Bowel regularity, a term often used casually, refers to the frequency, consistency, and ease of bowel movements. Achieving and maintaining regular bowel habits is a hallmark of a healthy digestive system. While dietary fiber, physical activity, and other lifestyle factors contribute to bowel regularity, hydration emerges as a central player in this intricate interplay.

1. Preventing Constipation: The most immediate impact of hydration on bowel regularity is its role in preventing constipation. Constipation, characterized by infrequent and hard-to-pass

stools, often arises from insufficient water intake. In the colon, water is absorbed from the stool, and when there is a deficit, the stool becomes dry and compacted, making it difficult to move through the intestines. Ensuring an ample supply of water helps maintain the proper consistency of stool, preventing constipation and promoting regular bowel movements.

2. Softening Stool: Water acts as a natural softener for stool, contributing to its pliability. Soft, well-hydrated stools are easier to pass through the colon, reducing the strain on the rectum and minimizing the likelihood of discomfort during bowel movements. This underscores the importance of hydration in ensuring that the digestive process culminates smoothly and without undue effort.

3. Promoting Regularity: Regular bowel movements are indicative of a well-functioning digestive system. Hydration plays a role in promoting the rhythmic contractions of the intestines, known as peristalsis, which propel stool forward. When the body is adequately hydrated, peristalsis operates efficiently, contributing to regular and predictable bowel movements. This regularity is essential for maintaining digestive health and preventing the development of chronic conditions such as irritable bowel syndrome (IBS) or inflammatory bowel disease (IBD).

4. Maintaining Gut Microbiome Balance: The gut microbiome, a complex community of microorganisms residing in the digestive tract, plays a crucial role in digestive and overall health. Adequate hydration supports the balance of this microbiome, fostering an environment conducive to the growth of beneficial bacteria. A harmonious gut microbiome contributes to optimal digestion and absorption of nutrients, further emphasizing the role of hydration in sustaining overall bowel health.

Factors Influencing Hydration Needs:

While the importance of hydration in supporting bowel regularity is clear, individual hydration needs can vary based on various factors. Understanding these factors allows individuals to tailor their hydration practices to meet their specific requirements:

1. Body Weight: The larger the body mass, the higher the water requirement. Individuals with higher body weight generally need more water to support various physiological functions, including digestion and bowel regularity.

2. Physical Activity: Exercise increases water loss through sweating, necessitating additional fluid intake to compensate for the loss. Staying hydrated is especially crucial for individuals engaged in regular physical activity, as dehydration can contribute to constipation and gastrointestinal discomfort.

3. Climate and Environment: Hot and humid climates, as well as high altitudes, can increase the body's water needs. In such conditions, individuals should be mindful of staying adequately hydrated to support digestive processes.

4. Dietary Habits: Certain foods, such as salty or spicy dishes, may increase thirst and, consequently, the need for hydration. Additionally, a diet rich in fruits and vegetables contributes to overall water intake, as these foods often have a high water content.

5. Medical Conditions: Certain medical conditions, such as diabetes or kidney disease, can affect water balance in the body. Individuals with these conditions may have specific hydration requirements and should consult healthcare professionals for personalized guidance.

Dehydration: A Disruptor of Digestive Harmony:

Conversely, inadequate hydration can disrupt the delicate balance of the digestive system, leading to a cascade of effects that compromise bowel regularity and overall digestive health:

1. Constipation: As mentioned earlier, dehydration is a common culprit in the development of constipation. When the body lacks sufficient water, the colon absorbs more water from the stool, resulting in dry and hardened feces that are difficult to pass.

2. Impaired Nutrient Absorption: Water is essential for the absorption of nutrients in the digestive tract. Dehydration can hinder this process, potentially leading to nutrient deficiencies and compromising overall health.

3. Increased Risk of Gastrointestinal Disorders: Chronic dehydration is associated with an increased risk of gastrointestinal disorders, including peptic ulcers and gastritis. The delicate mucosal lining of the digestive tract relies on adequate hydration for protection against irritants and pathogens.

4. Disruption of Gut Microbiome: The gut microbiome thrives in a hydrated environment. Dehydration can alter the composition of the microbiome, favoring the growth of harmful bacteria and compromising the balance essential for digestive health.

5. Electrolyte Imbalance: Electrolytes, such as sodium and potassium, play a crucial role in maintaining the balance of fluids in and around cells. Dehydration can disrupt electrolyte balance, impacting the function of muscles, including those in the digestive tract.

Practical Tips for Hydration and Digestive Health:

Understanding the integral connection between hydration and bowel regularity allows individuals to adopt practical strategies for maintaining optimal digestive health. Here are some tips to ensure adequate hydration and support regular bowel movements:

1. Water as the Primary Beverage: Make water the primary beverage of choice. While other beverages can contribute to overall fluid intake, water remains the purest and most effective hydrating option.

2. Consistent Water Intake Throughout the Day: Spread water intake evenly throughout the day. Sipping water consistently helps maintain hydration levels and supports ongoing digestive processes.

3. Monitor Urine Color: Pay attention to urine color as an indicator of hydration status. Pale yellow urine generally indicates adequate hydration, while dark yellow or amber urine may signal dehydration.

4. Consider Fluid-Rich Foods: Include fluid-rich foods in the diet, such as fruits and vegetables with high water content. This not only contributes to hydration but also provides essential nutrients and dietary fiber that support digestive health.

5. Hydrate Before, During, and After Exercise: Be mindful of hydration needs during physical activity. Hydrate before, during, and after exercise to compensate for fluid loss through sweating.

6. Limit Dehydrating Substances: Limit the consumption of substances that can contribute to dehydration, such as caffeine and alcohol. These beverages have diuretic effects and can increase urine production.

7. Create Hydration Habits: Establish hydration habits by incorporating water consumption into daily routines. Whether it's having a glass of water upon waking, before meals, or during work breaks, creating consistent habits fosters ongoing hydration.

8. Listen to Thirst Signals: Pay attention to the body's thirst signals. Thirst is a natural mechanism that indicates the need for fluid intake. Responding promptly to thirst helps maintain hydration balance.

Conclusion:

In the intricate dance of bodily functions, the power of hydration takes center stage, particularly in the realm of digestive health. Its influence extends beyond quenching thirst, reaching into the depths of the gastrointestinal tract, where it shapes the consistency of stool, facilitates nutrient absorption, and supports the harmonious functioning of the digestive system.

Understanding the symbiotic relationship between hydration and bowel regularity empowers individuals to make conscious choices that nurture digestive well-being. Whether through consistent water intake, mindful dietary choices, or attentive responses to the body's signals, prioritizing hydration is a foundational step towards maintaining optimal digestive health.

In the relentless pursuit of a balanced and vibrant life, acknowledging the power of hydration is akin to recognizing the conductor's baton in the symphony of well-being. It orchestrates the digestive processes with finesse, ensuring that the digestive system operates in seamless harmony. As we raise our glasses to the elixir of life, let us also toast to the enduring partnership between hydration and digestive vitality, a partnership that underscores the profound connection between our daily choices and the intricate dance of our internal rhythms.

CHAPTER SIX
Lifestyle Modifications for a Healthy Gut

The gut, often referred to as the "second brain," is a complex ecosystem that plays a pivotal role in maintaining overall health. A healthy gut is essential for optimal digestion, nutrient absorption, and immune function. Emerging research suggests that the gut also influences mental health, metabolism, and various systemic functions. In this exploration, we delve into the intricate web of lifestyle modifications that contribute to a healthy gut, encompassing dietary choices, physical activity, stress management, sleep hygiene, and the avoidance of detrimental habits.

Dietary Choices: The Foundation of Gut Health

Dietary habits exert a profound influence on the composition and function of the gut microbiome—the vast community of microorganisms residing in the digestive tract. A diverse and balanced diet provides the necessary nutrients for both the host (you) and the microbiome, fostering an environment conducive to gut health.

1. Fiber-Rich Foods: Dietary fiber, found in fruits, vegetables, whole grains, legumes, nuts, and seeds, is a cornerstone of gut health. Fiber acts as a prebiotic, nourishing beneficial bacteria in the gut. It adds bulk to the stool, supports regular bowel movements, and contributes to a thriving microbiome. Embracing a colorful array of plant-based foods ensures a spectrum of fibers that cater to different types of gut bacteria.

2. Fermented Foods: Incorporating fermented foods into the diet introduces probiotics—live beneficial bacteria. Yogurt, kefir, sauerkraut, kimchi, miso, and tempeh are examples of fermented foods that contribute to gut health. Probiotics play a crucial role in maintaining the balance of the gut microbiome, supporting immune function, and aiding in the digestion of certain nutrients.

3. Prebiotic-Rich Foods: Prebiotics are non-digestible fibers that serve as fuel for beneficial bacteria in the gut. Foods rich in prebiotics include garlic, onions, leeks, asparagus, bananas, and Jerusalem artichokes. By including prebiotic-rich foods in the diet, individuals can create an environment that nurtures the growth of beneficial gut bacteria.

4. Hydration: Water is indispensable for digestion and overall gut health. It helps break down food, facilitates the absorption of nutrients, and supports the movement of stool through the

intestines. Maintaining adequate hydration is crucial for preventing constipation and promoting optimal digestive function.

5. Limiting Highly Processed Foods: Highly processed foods, often laden with additives, preservatives, and artificial sweeteners, can negatively impact gut health. These foods may disrupt the balance of the microbiome and contribute to inflammation in the digestive tract. Opting for whole, minimally processed foods is a fundamental step in supporting a healthy gut.

6. Moderating Sugar and Artificial Sweeteners: Excessive intake of sugar and artificial sweeteners has been linked to negative effects on gut health. High sugar consumption can promote the growth of harmful bacteria, while certain artificial sweeteners may alter the composition of the microbiome. Moderation in sweetener intake, along with an emphasis on natural sugars from fruits, contributes to a healthier gut environment.

Physical Activity: Nourishing the Gut through Movement

Physical activity is not only beneficial for cardiovascular health and weight management but also plays a role in supporting a healthy gut. Exercise influences the composition and diversity of the gut microbiome and contributes to overall digestive well-being.

1. Promoting Gut Motility: Regular physical activity stimulates the muscles of the digestive tract, promoting gut motility. The rhythmic contractions of the intestines, known as peristalsis, are enhanced with exercise, facilitating the movement of stool through the digestive system. This can contribute to regular bowel movements and help prevent constipation.

2. Influencing Gut Microbiome Diversity: Exercise has been associated with increased gut microbiome diversity—a key indicator of gut health. A diverse microbiome is more resilient to disturbances, supports immune function, and contributes to the efficient breakdown of dietary fibers. Engaging in a variety of physical activities, from aerobic exercise to resistance training, enhances microbiome diversity.

3. Reducing Inflammation: Chronic inflammation in the gut is implicated in various digestive disorders. Regular exercise has anti-inflammatory effects that extend to the gastrointestinal tract. By reducing systemic inflammation, exercise helps create a favorable environment for a healthy gut.

4. Supporting Weight Management: Maintaining a healthy weight is crucial for gut health, as excess body weight has been linked to an increased risk of gastrointestinal conditions. Physical activity contributes to weight management, and its positive effects on metabolism and insulin sensitivity further support digestive health.

Stress Management: The Mind-Gut Connection

The intricate relationship between the mind and the gut is a burgeoning field of research known as the gut-brain axis. Stress, anxiety, and other emotional factors can significantly influence gut function, emphasizing the importance of stress management in maintaining a healthy gut.

1. Mindful Eating: Adopting mindful eating practices contributes to better digestion. Eating in a relaxed environment, savoring each bite, and paying attention to hunger and fullness cues can positively impact gut function. Mindful eating also encourages the consumption of a varied and balanced diet, supporting overall gut health.

2. Stress Reduction Techniques: Chronic stress can lead to changes in gut motility, blood flow, and immune function. Incorporating stress reduction techniques, such as deep breathing, meditation, yoga, or tai chi, can mitigate the impact of stress on the gut. These practices contribute to a calmer nervous system and foster a more resilient gut environment.

3. Adequate Sleep: Quality sleep is integral to overall well-being, including gut health. Sleep disturbances, such as insufficient or disrupted sleep, can influence the gut-brain axis and contribute to gastrointestinal issues. Prioritizing good sleep hygiene, including consistent sleep schedules and creating a conducive sleep environment, supports both mental and digestive health.

Avoidance of Detrimental Habits: Protecting the Gut Terrain

Certain lifestyle habits can compromise gut health and disrupt the delicate balance of the microbiome. Recognizing and avoiding these detrimental habits is pivotal in promoting a resilient and flourishing gut environment.

1. Excessive Use of Antibiotics: Antibiotics, while crucial for treating bacterial infections, can also disrupt the balance of the gut microbiome. Excessive or unnecessary use of antibiotics may lead to an overgrowth of harmful bacteria and a reduction in beneficial bacteria. When prescribed antibiotics, it is essential to follow healthcare provider recommendations and consider probiotic supplementation to support microbiome recovery.

2. Overconsumption of Alcohol: Excessive alcohol intake can have detrimental effects on the gut lining and microbiome. It may lead to inflammation, increased permeability of the intestinal

barrier (leaky gut), and alterations in the composition of gut bacteria. Moderation in alcohol consumption is advisable for maintaining gut health.

3. Cigarette Smoking: Cigarette smoking has been linked to various gastrointestinal disorders, including inflammatory bowel disease (IBD) and peptic ulcers. Smoking can disrupt the protective mucosal layer of the digestive tract and contribute to inflammation. Quitting smoking is a crucial step in preserving gut health and overall well-being.

4. Inadequate Hydration: Dehydration can compromise gut function, leading to constipation and other digestive issues. Insufficient water intake hinders the smooth passage of stool through the

intestines and may contribute to the development of gastrointestinal conditions. Prioritizing adequate hydration is essential for maintaining optimal gut health.

5. Inconsistent Meal Timing: Erratic meal timing or skipping meals can disrupt the circadian rhythm of the digestive system. Regular and consistent meal patterns support the synchronization of digestive processes, optimizing nutrient absorption and promoting gut health.

Conclusion: Cultivating a Lifestyle for Gut Resilience

The quest for a healthy gut transcends mere dietary choices; it encompasses a holistic approach to lifestyle that nurtures the intricate balance within the digestive system. From the foods we consume to the way we move, manage stress, and prioritize sleep, every facet of our lifestyle contributes to the flourishing ecosystem of the gut.

Understanding the symbiotic relationship between lifestyle and gut health empowers individuals to make informed choices that resonate with their unique needs. Embracing a plant-rich, fiber-filled diet, incorporating regular physical activity, practicing stress management techniques, ensuring adequate sleep, and avoiding detrimental habits collectively create an environment where the gut can thrive.

In the tapestry of well-being, the gut emerges as a central thread, woven intricately with the choices we make each day. As we navigate the complexities of modern life, fostering a healthy gut becomes a deliberate and empowering endeavor—one that not only influences digestive health but ripples across the entire spectrum of wellness.

In the canvas of our lives, let us paint a portrait of gut resilience—a portrait that reflects the wisdom of mindful choices, the vitality of nourishing foods, and the harmony of a lifestyle attuned to the needs of our second brain. With each step towards a gut-friendly lifestyle, we embark on a journey of self-care, recognizing that the choices we make today shape the landscape of our well-being tomorrow.

CHAPTER SEVEN
Exercise and Constipation: Finding the Right Balance

In the intricate dance of bodily functions, the relationship between exercise and digestive health is a dynamic interplay that often takes center stage. Regular physical activity is celebrated for its myriad benefits, from cardiovascular health to weight management and mental well-being. However, within this harmonious symphony, constipation emerges as a common concern that can disrupt the rhythm of daily life. In this exploration, we delve into the complex association between exercise and constipation, seeking to understand the mechanisms at play, dispel common myths, and provide practical insights into finding the right balance for digestive harmony.

The Interconnected Systems: Unraveling the Link

The digestive system and the musculoskeletal system, which governs movement and exercise, are intricately connected. The communication between these systems involves a network of nerves, hormones, and physiological responses. Understanding how exercise influences digestion requires a closer look at the mechanisms that underlie this interconnectedness.

Peristalsis, the rhythmic contractions of the muscles in the digestive tract, propels food and waste through the intestines. Exercise, particularly aerobic activities like walking, jogging, or cycling, stimulates peristalsis. The mechanical movement associated with these exercises helps move stool through the intestines, potentially alleviating constipation.

Exercise increases blood flow to various organs, including the digestive organs. This heightened blood flow supports the efficient transport of nutrients and oxygen to the intestines. Improved blood circulation can enhance the overall function of the digestive system, contributing to regular bowel movements.

The gut microbiome, a complex community of microorganisms in the digestive tract, plays a crucial role in digestive health. Regular exercise has been associated with positive changes in the composition of the gut microbiome. A diverse and balanced microbiome contributes to optimal digestion and may play a role in preventing constipation.

Stress, whether acute or chronic, can impact digestion and contribute to constipation. Exercise is a well-known stress-reducer, releasing endorphins and promoting a sense of well-being. By mitigating stress levels, exercise indirectly supports digestive health and may help prevent constipation.

Exercise Myths and Constipation: Dispelling Misconceptions

While exercise is generally beneficial for digestive health, several myths and misconceptions surround the relationship between physical activity and constipation. Dispelling these myths is crucial for understanding the nuanced dynamics at play:

1. Myth: Exercise Always Causes Dehydration and Constipation: Some believe that exercise leads to dehydration, contributing to constipation. While it's true that dehydration can lead to constipation, moderate exercise does not necessarily cause dehydration. In fact, staying hydrated during exercise is essential for supporting digestive processes.

2. Myth: Only Intense Exercise Affects Bowel Habits: There is a common belief that only high-intensity or vigorous exercise influences bowel habits. However, even moderate and low-intensity activities, such as walking or gentle yoga, can have a positive impact on digestion. The key is to find a balance that suits individual fitness levels and preferences.

3. Myth: Sedentary Lifestyle Alleviates Constipation: Some individuals may assume that a sedentary lifestyle is the antidote to constipation. However, lack of physical activity can contribute to sluggish bowel movements. Incorporating regular, moderate exercise is generally more conducive to maintaining healthy bowel habits.

4. Myth: Abdominal Exercises Alone Solve Constipation: While exercises that engage the abdominal muscles can contribute to digestive health, solely focusing on abdominal exercises is not a comprehensive solution to constipation. A holistic approach that includes a variety of exercises and lifestyle factors is essential for optimal digestive function.

Finding the Right Balance: Tailoring Exercise for Digestive Harmony

Optimizing the relationship between exercise and constipation involves finding the right balance based on individual factors, preferences, and health conditions. Here are practical insights into tailoring exercise for digestive harmony:

1. Incorporate Regular Physical Activity: Consistency is key when it comes to the benefits of exercise for digestive health. Aim for at least 150 minutes of moderate-intensity aerobic exercise per week, as recommended by health guidelines. This can include activities such as brisk walking, cycling, or swimming.

2. Diversify Your Exercise Routine: Engage in a variety of exercises that incorporate different muscle groups. This diversity not only enhances overall fitness but also stimulates different aspects of the digestive system. Include aerobic exercises, strength training, and flexibility exercises in your routine.

3. Listen to Your Body: Pay attention to how your body responds to different types and intensities of exercise. Some individuals may find that moderate-intensity activities like walking or jogging positively influence bowel habits, while others may prefer activities like yoga or swimming.

4. Stay Hydrated: Adequate hydration is crucial for digestive health. Drink water before, during, and after exercise to prevent dehydration. Dehydration can lead to harder stools and contribute to constipation. The color of urine can serve as a simple indicator of hydration status—pale yellow indicates adequate hydration.

5. Mind Your Pre-Exercise Nutrition: Consider your pre-exercise nutrition, especially if you plan to engage in more intense activities. Eating a balanced meal or snack that includes carbohydrates, protein, and a moderate amount of fiber before exercise can provide energy and support digestive processes.

6. Be Mindful of Intense Exercise: Intense or high-intensity exercise may influence bowel habits differently for each individual. For some, vigorous exercise may stimulate bowel movements, while for others, it may cause temporary changes. Pay attention to your body's responses and adjust the intensity and timing of exercise accordingly.

7. Consider Timing Around Meals: Some individuals find that light exercise after meals, such as a short walk, aids digestion. Experiment with the timing of your exercise routine to determine what works best for your digestive comfort. Avoid intense exercise immediately after large meals.

8. Explore Relaxation Exercises: Incorporate relaxation exercises, such as deep breathing or gentle yoga, into your routine. These activities can help manage stress, which, in turn, supports

digestive health. Chronic stress can contribute to constipation, so finding ways to relax is beneficial.

9. Consult with Healthcare Professionals: If constipation persists despite lifestyle modifications, it's essential to consult with healthcare professionals. Underlying medical conditions or medications could be contributing to digestive issues. A comprehensive evaluation can help tailor recommendations to individual needs.

Addressing Constipation Through Comprehensive Lifestyle Changes

While exercise is a valuable component of a healthy lifestyle, addressing constipation often requires a multifaceted approach that extends beyond physical activity. Here are additional lifestyle modifications that can complement exercise for digestive well-being:

1. Prioritize Dietary Fiber: A diet rich in fiber is essential for promoting regular bowel movements. Include a variety of fruits, vegetables, whole grains, legumes, nuts, and seeds in your diet. Fiber adds bulk to the stool, softens it, and supports the smooth passage of waste through the intestines.

2. Hydrate Adequately: Proper hydration is crucial for preventing constipation. Water softens the stool, making it easier to pass through the digestive tract. Aim to drink enough water throughout the day, and consider herbal teas or infused water for additional hydration.

3. Establish Regular Meal Patterns: Consistent meal patterns contribute to the synchronization of digestive processes. Aim to have meals at regular times each day, and avoid skipping meals, which can disrupt the natural rhythm of the digestive system.

4. Include Probiotic-Rich Foods: Probiotics, beneficial bacteria that support gut health, can be found in fermented foods such as yogurt, kefir, sauerkraut, and kimchi. Including these foods in your diet can contribute to a balanced gut microbiome.

5. Manage Stress: Chronic stress can contribute to constipation. Incorporate stress management techniques into your routine, such as mindfulness meditation, progressive muscle relaxation, or activities that bring joy and relaxation.

6. Prioritize Adequate Sleep: Quality sleep is integral to overall well-being, including digestive health. Ensure that you get enough restful sleep each night, as sleep disturbances can impact the gut-brain axis and contribute to constipation.

7. Limit Processed Foods and Stimulants: Highly processed foods, especially those low in fiber, can contribute to constipation. Additionally, excessive consumption of caffeinated beverages and certain stimulants may have a laxative effect but can also lead to dependency. Moderation is key.

8. Consider Dietary Modifications: In some cases, specific dietary modifications may be beneficial. For example, some individuals may find relief from constipation by limiting dairy or identifying specific trigger foods. Consulting with a registered dietitian can provide personalized guidance.

Conclusion: Navigating the Path to Digestive Well-Being

In the intricate landscape of digestive health, the role of exercise in preventing or alleviating constipation is a vital thread. Understanding the interplay between exercise, lifestyle factors, and digestive function empowers individuals to make informed choices that contribute to overall well-being.

As we navigate the nuanced relationship between exercise and constipation, it becomes clear that a personalized and holistic approach is key. Tailoring exercise routines to individual preferences, considering overall lifestyle factors, and being attuned to the body's signals create a roadmap for digestive harmony.

In the grand symphony of health, where each note contributes to the melody of well-being, finding the right balance between exercise and constipation is a nuanced art. It requires listening to the body's cues, making conscious lifestyle choices, and recognizing that the journey to digestive well-being is a dynamic and evolving process.

As we lace up our sneakers, roll out our yoga mats, or embark on a brisk walk, let us embrace the synergy between movement and digestion. In the rhythmic cadence of exercise, we find not only the joy of physical vitality but also the potential for a well-balanced and harmonious digestive system. With each step, we embark on a journey towards a vibrant and resilient digestive terrain—a journey where the dance of exercise and the rhythm of digestion intertwine, creating a symphony of health that resonates throughout the body and enriches the tapestry of our lives.

CHAPTER EIGHT

Supplements and Remedies for Effective Fiber Intake

In the ever-evolving landscape of nutrition and wellness, the role of dietary fiber stands as a stalwart pillar in promoting digestive health and overall well-being. While a balanced and varied diet rich in fruits, vegetables, whole grains, legumes, nuts, and seeds is the ideal way to meet fiber needs, there are instances where individuals may seek additional support through supplements and remedies. This comprehensive exploration delves into the diverse array of fiber supplements, natural remedies, and lifestyle strategies designed to enhance fiber intake, providing insights into their efficacy, considerations for usage, and their place in the broader context of a healthy lifestyle.

Despite the well-established benefits of dietary fiber, many individuals struggle to meet the recommended daily intake. Factors such as busy lifestyles, dietary preferences, and certain medical conditions can contribute to what is often referred to as the "fiber gap." The recommended daily intake of fiber varies by age and gender, but, in general, adults are advised to consume between 25 to 38 grams of fiber per day, according to dietary guidelines.

Addressing the fiber gap is crucial, as inadequate fiber intake is associated with various health concerns, including constipation, digestive issues, and an increased risk of chronic diseases such as cardiovascular disease and certain cancers. To bridge this gap, individuals may turn to fiber supplements and natural remedies as practical solutions to enhance their overall fiber intake.

Fiber Supplements: Exploring Options and Considerations

Fiber supplements are concentrated forms of fiber that come in various formulations, including powders, capsules, chewable tablets, and gummies. These supplements offer a convenient way to boost fiber intake, but it's essential to understand the different types of fiber supplements, how they work, and potential considerations for usage.

1. Psyllium Husk: Psyllium husk is a soluble fiber derived from the seeds of the Plantago ovata plant. It is a key ingredient in many fiber supplements and is known for its ability to absorb water and form a gel-like substance. Psyllium husk supplements, available in powder or capsule form, are often used to relieve constipation and promote bowel regularity.

2. Methylcellulose: Methylcellulose is a synthetic, non-fermentable soluble fiber that is often used in fiber supplements. It has water-holding properties and adds bulk to the stool, similar to psyllium

husk. Methylcellulose supplements may be suitable for individuals who are allergic to psyllium or prefer a non-plant-based option.

3. Inulin: Inulin is a soluble fiber found in certain plant foods, such as chicory root, garlic, and onions. It is also used as an ingredient in some fiber supplements. Inulin is a prebiotic, meaning it supports the growth of beneficial bacteria in the gut. While generally well-tolerated, inulin supplements may cause gas or bloating in some individuals.

4. Glucomannan: Glucomannan is a water-soluble fiber extracted from the root of the konjac plant. It has a high water-holding capacity and is often used as a thickening agent in food

products and as a dietary supplement. Glucomannan supplements are known for their potential to promote a feeling of fullness and support weight management.

5. Wheat Dextrin: Wheat dextrin is a soluble fiber derived from wheat starch. It is commonly used as an additive in processed foods and is also available as a fiber supplement. Wheat dextrin supplements may be a suitable option for those looking to increase their fiber intake.

Considerations for Using Fiber Supplements:

While fiber supplements can be a valuable tool in meeting daily fiber goals, it's essential to approach their usage with considerations for individual needs and potential effects:

1. Start Gradually: Introduce fiber supplements gradually to allow the digestive system to adjust. Sudden increases in fiber intake can lead to bloating, gas, or stomach cramps. Begin with a lower dose and gradually increase as tolerated.

2. Stay Hydrated: Fiber supplements absorb water, so it's crucial to drink plenty of fluids when using them. Adequate hydration helps prevent constipation and supports the smooth passage of fiber through the digestive tract.

3. Individual Tolerance: Different individuals may respond differently to various types of fiber supplements. It may be necessary to experiment with different options to find the one that is best tolerated and aligns with individual preferences.

4. Consider Underlying Conditions: Individuals with certain medical conditions, such as irritable bowel syndrome (IBS) or inflammatory bowel disease (IBD), should consult healthcare professionals before using fiber supplements. The type and amount of fiber that is well-tolerated can vary based on specific health conditions.

5. Read Labels Carefully: When choosing a fiber supplement, carefully read labels to understand the type of fiber it contains and any additional ingredients. Some supplements may contain added sugars, artificial sweeteners, or other additives that may not align with individual preferences.

6. Medication Interactions: Fiber supplements may interact with certain medications, affecting their absorption or efficacy. Individuals taking medications should consult healthcare professionals to ensure that fiber supplements do not interfere with their prescribed treatments.

7. Not a Replacement for Whole Foods: While fiber supplements can be a convenient option, they should not be viewed as a replacement for whole, fiber-rich foods. Whole foods provide a spectrum of nutrients, including vitamins, minerals, and antioxidants, which contribute to overall health.

Natural Remedies to Boost Fiber Intake: A Holistic Approach

In addition to fiber supplements, several natural remedies and lifestyle strategies can be incorporated to enhance overall fiber intake. These remedies emphasize whole, unprocessed foods and lifestyle choices that align with a holistic approach to well-being:

1. Chia Seeds: Chia seeds are tiny powerhouses of nutrition, rich in both soluble and insoluble fiber. When mixed with liquids, chia seeds form a gel-like consistency, making them a versatile addition to smoothies, yogurt, or oatmeal. Chia seeds provide not only fiber but also omega-3 fatty acids, antioxidants, and minerals.

2. Flaxseeds: Flaxseeds, whether ground or in oil form, are excellent sources of soluble and insoluble fiber. They also contain alpha-linolenic acid (ALA), a type of omega-3 fatty acid. Sprinkling ground flaxseeds on cereals, salads, or incorporating flaxseed oil into dressings are convenient ways to boost fiber intake.

3. Amaranth and Quinoa: Amaranth and quinoa are ancient grains that offer a notable amount of dietary fiber along with protein and essential nutrients. These grains can be used as alternatives to traditional grains in salads, soups, or as side dishes, contributing to a diversified fiber intake.

4. Vegetable Smoothies: Blending vegetables into smoothies is a tasty way to increase fiber intake. Leafy greens, carrots, beets, and other vegetables can be combined with fruits, yogurt, or plant-based milk to create nutrient-rich and fiber-packed beverages.

5. Prunes and Dried Fruits: Prunes, or dried plums, are well-known for their natural laxative effect. They contain both soluble and insoluble fiber, along with sorbitol, a natural sugar alcohol that can have a mild laxative effect. Dried fruits like apricots, figs, and raisins are also fiber-rich options.

6. Bran Cereals: Bran cereals, especially those made from wheat or oats, are concentrated sources of dietary fiber. Adding bran cereals to yogurt, milk, or incorporating them into recipes provides an easy and palatable way to increase fiber intake.

7. Beans and Legumes: Beans and legumes, including lentils, chickpeas, black beans, and kidney beans, are high-fiber foods that offer a plethora of health benefits. They can be added to soups, stews, salads, or used as a protein-rich base for various dishes.

8. Root Vegetables: Root vegetables like sweet potatoes, carrots, and beets are not only rich in fiber but also provide essential vitamins and minerals. Roasting or steaming these vegetables can enhance their natural flavors and nutritional content.

9. Whole Grains: Whole grains, such as brown rice, quinoa, barley, and whole wheat, are integral components of a fiber-rich diet. Substituting refined grains with their whole counterparts in meals like rice bowls, salads, and side dishes can significantly increase fiber intake.

Lifestyle Strategies for Optimal Fiber Intake:

In addition to incorporating fiber-rich foods and considering supplements and remedies, certain lifestyle strategies can further support the goal of achieving optimal fiber intake:

1. Meal Planning: Planning meals in advance allows individuals to include a variety of fiber-rich foods. Designing well-balanced meals that encompass fruits, vegetables, whole grains, and legumes helps ensure consistent fiber intake throughout the day.

2. Mindful Eating: Practicing mindful eating involves savoring each bite, paying attention to hunger and fullness cues, and avoiding distractions during meals. This approach supports healthier food choices and encourages the consumption of fiber-rich, nutrient-dense foods.

3. Hydration: Adequate hydration is crucial for the proper functioning of fiber in the digestive system. Water helps soften the stool, facilitating its movement through the intestines. Drinking water throughout the day is essential, especially when consuming a fiber-rich diet.

4. Regular Physical Activity: Physical activity stimulates bowel movements and contributes to overall digestive health. Engaging in regular exercise, whether it's walking, jogging, or other forms of aerobic activity, supports the natural rhythm of the digestive system.

5. Gradual Dietary Changes: When transitioning to a higher-fiber diet, making gradual changes allows the digestive system to adapt. Sudden increases in fiber intake may lead to digestive discomfort, and a gradual approach can help mitigate these effects.

6. Diversification of Fiber Sources: Embracing a diverse range of fiber sources ensures that individuals benefit from a spectrum of nutrients and fiber types. A colorful array of fruits, vegetables, whole grains, legumes, nuts, and seeds provides a broad spectrum of dietary fibers.

7. Individualized Approach: Recognizing that individual responses to fiber intake can vary, adopting an individualized approach is key. What works for one person may not work for another, and adjustments may be necessary based on personal preferences and tolerances.

Conclusion: Weaving Fiber into the Fabric of Wellness

In the quest for optimal digestive health and overall well-being, the role of fiber is woven into the very fabric of our dietary choices and lifestyle habits. While whole, fiber-rich foods remain the cornerstone of a healthy diet, supplements and remedies offer valuable support for those seeking to bridge the fiber gap or address specific dietary challenges.

As we navigate the diverse landscape of fiber supplements, natural remedies, and lifestyle strategies, it's essential to approach the journey with mindfulness, individualization, and a holistic perspective. The goal is not merely to meet a recommended daily intake but to cultivate a sustainable and enjoyable relationship with fiber, one that enhances the symphony of well-being in our daily lives.

In embracing the richness of fiber from various sources—be it the wholesome crunch of nuts, the earthy goodness of whole grains, or the vibrant hues of fruits and vegetables—we embark on a journey that transcends mere nutritional value. It becomes a journey of self-discovery, where the choices we make resonate not only with our digestive well-being but with the vitality of our entire being.

As we incorporate fiber supplements into our daily routines, sprinkle chia seeds on our morning yogurt, or savor the natural sweetness of dried fruits, let us do so with a sense of reverence for the intricacies of our bodies. In this symbiotic dance of nourishment and well-being, fiber emerges as a steadfast partner—a gentle guide that supports us on our quest for vitality, resilience, and the joy that comes from weaving wellness into the very fabric of our lives.

CHAPTER NINE

Overcoming Common Challenges in Fiber Therapy for Constipation

In the realm of digestive health, constipation stands as a common and often vexing concern that can significantly impact one's quality of life. Amid the myriad approaches to address constipation, fiber therapy emerges as a cornerstone—a tried-and-true method that aims to promote regular bowel movements and alleviate discomfort. However, the landscape of fiber therapy is not without its challenges. In this comprehensive exploration, we delve into the nuances of overcoming common obstacles in fiber therapy for constipation, understanding the intricacies of dietary fiber, unraveling the factors that contribute to constipation, and charting a course toward effective and personalized solutions.

Common Challenges in Fiber Therapy for Constipation:

1. Inadequate Fiber Intake: One of the primary challenges in fiber therapy is inadequate fiber intake. Many individuals do not meet the recommended daily intake of fiber, which varies based on age, gender, and individual needs. The recommended range is typically between 25 to 38 grams per day for adults.

Solution: Gradual Increase in Fiber Intake: Addressing inadequate fiber intake involves a gradual increase in the consumption of fiber-rich foods. Abrupt changes in fiber intake can lead to digestive discomfort, so incorporating fiber gradually allows the digestive system to adapt.

2. Limited Variety of Fiber Sources: Another challenge is the reliance on a limited variety of fiber sources. Some individuals may consume fiber primarily from one source, such as whole grains, while neglecting other sources like fruits, vegetables, nuts, and seeds.

Solution: Diversification of Fiber Intake: Diversifying fiber sources ensures a broader spectrum of nutrients and fiber types. Including a variety of fruits, vegetables, whole grains, legumes, nuts, and seeds in the diet provides different types of fiber with unique health benefits.

3. Low Fluid Intake: Adequate fluid intake is essential for the effectiveness of fiber therapy. Fiber absorbs water, and insufficient hydration can lead to a situation where fiber becomes more likely to cause constipation instead of relieving it.

Solution: Hydration Awareness: Emphasizing the importance of staying hydrated is crucial in fiber therapy. Individuals should be mindful of their fluid intake, especially when increasing fiber consumption, to prevent dehydration and promote optimal stool consistency.

4. Individual Tolerance Variability: The response to increased fiber intake can vary widely among individuals. Some may experience bloating, gas, or abdominal discomfort, particularly when introducing new fiber sources.

Solution: Individualized Approach: Recognizing that individual tolerance to fiber varies, an individualized approach is key. Experimenting with different fiber sources and observing how the body responds allows for the identification of well-tolerated options.

5. Impact of Dietary Preferences: Dietary preferences, including vegetarianism, veganism, or specific food intolerances, can impact the feasibility and sustainability of fiber therapy. Limited food choices may make it challenging to achieve the recommended fiber intake.

Solution: Tailoring Fiber Sources to Preferences: Tailoring fiber sources to align with dietary preferences is essential. For example, plant-based diets can include a variety of legumes, nuts, seeds, and whole grains to meet fiber needs while accommodating dietary choices.

6. Lack of Awareness About Fiber Content: Many individuals may lack awareness of the fiber content in different foods. Without this knowledge, it becomes challenging to make informed choices that support fiber therapy.

Solution: Education and Awareness: Education about the fiber content of various foods is a fundamental aspect of overcoming this challenge. Providing information and resources that help individuals identify high-fiber foods empowers them to make intentional dietary choices.

7. Sedentary Lifestyle: A sedentary lifestyle can contribute to constipation, and relying solely on fiber therapy without addressing overall physical activity levels may limit its effectiveness.

Solution: Incorporating Physical Activity: Encouraging regular physical activity supports the natural movement of the digestive tract and complements the effects of fiber therapy. Simple activities like walking or jogging can contribute to overall digestive health.

8. Chronic Conditions and Medications: Underlying medical conditions, such as irritable bowel syndrome (IBS) or certain medications, may impact the effectiveness of fiber therapy. In some cases, these conditions may require additional considerations and personalized approaches.

Solution: Consultation with Healthcare Professionals: Seeking guidance from healthcare professionals is crucial when constipation is associated with underlying medical conditions or medications. They can provide personalized recommendations and ensure that fiber therapy aligns with individual health needs.

Strategies for Overcoming Challenges in Fiber Therapy:

1. Gradual Increase in Fiber Intake: Overcoming the challenge of inadequate fiber intake involves a gradual and systematic approach. Individuals can start by adding one high-fiber food item to each meal and gradually increasing fiber-rich choices over time.

2. Diversification of Fiber Sources: To address the limitation of fiber sources, individuals can create a diverse meal plan that includes a variety of fruits, vegetables, whole grains, legumes, nuts, and seeds. Experimenting with new recipes and exploring different cuisines can contribute to a varied and enjoyable diet.

3. Hydration Awareness: Staying hydrated is crucial for the effectiveness of fiber therapy. Individuals can cultivate awareness of their fluid intake by carrying a water bottle, setting reminders to drink water, and choosing hydrating foods like water-rich fruits and vegetables.

4. Individualized Approach: Recognizing the variability in individual tolerance requires an individualized approach to fiber therapy. Keeping a food diary, monitoring symptoms, and making adjustments based on personal responses can help tailor fiber intake to individual needs.

5. Tailoring Fiber Sources to Preferences: Aligning fiber sources with dietary preferences involves exploring plant-based options that fit within chosen dietary frameworks. For example, incorporating a variety of legumes, nuts, seeds, and whole grains into vegetarian or vegan diets can enhance fiber intake.

6. Education and Awareness: Overcoming the lack of awareness about fiber content involves education and resources. Providing information about the fiber content of common foods, offering recipe ideas, and promoting nutrition labels as tools for informed choices contribute to increased awareness.

7. Incorporating Physical Activity: To address the impact of a sedentary lifestyle, individuals can incorporate physical activity into their daily routines. Simple activities like walking, cycling, or engaging in regular exercise routines support overall digestive health and enhance the effectiveness of fiber therapy.

8. Consultation with Healthcare Professionals: When dealing with chronic conditions or medications that may impact fiber therapy, seeking guidance from healthcare professionals is paramount. Healthcare providers can offer personalized recommendations, adjust treatment plans, and address specific health concerns.

Holistic Approaches to Fiber Therapy:

1. Whole-Food Emphasis: Emphasizing whole foods as sources of fiber is a holistic approach that aligns with overall health and nutrition. Whole foods provide not only fiber but also a spectrum of nutrients, including vitamins, minerals, antioxidants, and phytochemicals.

2. Mindful Eating Practices: Mindful eating practices, such as savoring each bite, paying attention to hunger and fullness cues, and avoiding distractions during meals, complement fiber therapy. These practices encourage a healthier relationship with food and support intentional dietary choices.

3. Balanced Nutrition: Balancing nutrition involves considering the overall nutrient composition of meals. Combining fiber-rich foods with sources of protein, healthy fats, and a variety of vitamins and minerals contributes to a well-rounded and nutritionally dense diet.

4. Stress Management: Stress management is integral to digestive health, and chronic stress can contribute to constipation. Incorporating stress-reducing practices such as meditation, deep breathing exercises, or engaging in activities that bring joy and relaxation supports overall well-being.

5. Regular Monitoring and Adjustment: Regularly monitoring symptoms and adjusting dietary choices based on individual responses are key components of holistic fiber therapy. This ongoing process allows individuals to fine-tune their approach, ensuring sustained benefits.

Conclusion: Navigating the Path to Digestive Harmony

In the intricate dance of dietary choices, lifestyle habits, and individual responses, overcoming common challenges in fiber therapy for constipation becomes a journey of self-discovery and intentional well-being. As we navigate this path, it becomes evident that constipation is not a one-size-fits-all concern, and fiber therapy is not a uniform solution. Instead, it is a personalized and holistic approach that requires mindfulness, flexibility, and a nuanced understanding of the body's signals.

In embracing the principles of fiber therapy, we weave a tapestry of digestive harmony—a tapestry where the vibrant hues of fruits and vegetables, the wholesome crunch of nuts and seeds, and the nourishing richness of whole grains create a symphony of well-being. It is a journey where the complexities of constipation are met with the simplicity and efficacy of dietary fiber—a journey that transcends the confines of a mere therapeutic approach and becomes a way of life.

As we savor the flavors of fiber-rich meals, relish the crispness of fresh produce, and celebrate the nourishing power of plant-based foods, let us do so with a sense of empowerment. In the realm of fiber therapy, where challenges are met with solutions, and individualized approaches pave the way, we find not only relief from constipation but a profound connection to the innate wisdom of our bodies.

In this exploration of overcoming common challenges in fiber therapy, let us remember that the journey is as significant as the destination. It is a journey that invites us to tune into the needs of our bodies, embrace the diversity of fiber sources, and cultivate a lifestyle that supports not just digestive health but the flourishing vitality of our entire being. As we navigate this path, may we find joy in the simplicity of fiber-rich choices, revel in the resilience of our digestive systems, and embark on a journey toward enduring well-being—one fiber-filled choice at a time.

CHAPTER TEN
Sustaining Long-Term Gut Wellness: Maintenance Strategies

In the intricate tapestry of human health, the gut plays a pivotal role, serving as a central hub for digestion, nutrient absorption, and interactions with the immune system. Achieving and sustaining long-term gut wellness is a multifaceted journey that involves a harmonious interplay of dietary choices, lifestyle habits, and proactive measures. This comprehensive exploration delves into the dynamic landscape of gut health, unraveling the intricacies of the gut microbiome, understanding the factors that contribute to gut imbalances, and offering evidence-based maintenance strategies for nurturing enduring gut wellness.

The Gut Microbiome: A Microscopic Ecosystem

At the heart of gut wellness lies the microbiome—a complex and diverse community of microorganisms that inhabit the digestive tract. Comprising bacteria, viruses, fungi, and other microbes, the gut microbiome is a dynamic ecosystem that influences various aspects of health, from digestion and metabolism to immune function and mental well-being.

The gut microbiome is primarily composed of bacteria, with thousands of different species coexisting in a delicate balance. Bacterial diversity is a key indicator of a healthy microbiome, as different species play distinct roles in maintaining gut function.

Microbes in the gut aid in the breakdown of complex carbohydrates, the fermentation of dietary fibers, and the production of essential nutrients. This symbiotic relationship between the host and its microbial inhabitants is essential for optimal digestive function.

The gut is a critical interface between the external environment and the immune system. The microbiome plays a crucial role in training and modulating the immune system, helping to distinguish between harmful pathogens and beneficial microbes.

Microbes in the gut contribute to the synthesis of bioactive compounds, including short-chain fatty acids (SCFAs) and certain vitamins. These compounds have far-reaching effects on metabolic health, inflammation, and overall well-being.

Factors Influencing Gut Health

Achieving long-term gut wellness requires an understanding of the factors that can influence the delicate balance of the gut microbiome. Several elements, ranging from dietary choices to lifestyle habits, can impact gut health:

1. Dietary Factors:

   - Fiber Intake: A diet rich in fiber promotes the growth of beneficial bacteria in the gut. Whole plant foods, such as fruits, vegetables, whole grains, legumes, and nuts, provide a diverse array of fibers that nourish the microbiome.

   - Probiotics and Fermented Foods: Probiotics, found in fermented foods like yogurt, kefir, sauerkraut, and kimchi, introduce beneficial live bacteria to the gut, supporting microbial diversity.

   - Prebiotics: Prebiotics are non-digestible fibers that serve as food for beneficial bacteria. Foods like garlic, onions, leeks, and bananas contain prebiotics that foster a healthy gut environment.

2. Lifestyle Habits:

   - Physical Activity: Regular exercise has been associated with a more diverse and resilient gut microbiome. Physical activity promotes gut motility and the release of compounds that positively impact microbial composition.

   - Sleep Quality: Adequate and quality sleep is essential for overall well-being, including gut health. Disruptions in sleep patterns have been linked to changes in the gut microbiome and increased inflammation.

3. Stress and Mental Health:

- Stress Management: Chronic stress can negatively impact gut health by influencing the composition of the microbiome and contributing to inflammation. Stress management techniques such as mindfulness, meditation, and relaxation exercises are beneficial.

- Gut-Brain Axis: The bidirectional communication between the gut and the brain, known as the gut-brain axis, plays a crucial role in mental health. A balanced and healthy gut contributes to emotional well-being and cognitive function.

4. Antibiotic Use:

- Impact on Microbiome: Antibiotics, while crucial for treating infections, can have a significant impact on the gut microbiome. They may lead to a temporary disruption in microbial balance, emphasizing the importance of targeted and judicious antibiotic use.

5. Environmental Exposures:

- Chemical Exposures: Certain environmental factors, including exposure to pesticides, pollutants, and other chemicals, may influence the gut microbiome. Minimizing exposure to harmful substances supports gut health.

6. Hydration:

- Importance of Water: Adequate hydration is fundamental for digestive health. Water supports the movement of food through the digestive tract, preventing constipation and promoting a healthy gut environment.

Maintenance Strategies for Long-Term Gut Wellness

With an understanding of the intricacies surrounding gut health and the factors that contribute to its delicate balance, adopting evidence-based maintenance strategies becomes paramount for sustained well-being. These strategies encompass a holistic approach, addressing dietary, lifestyle, and environmental aspects of gut health.

1. Prioritize a Plant-Rich Diet:

- Diverse Fiber Sources: A plant-rich diet that includes a variety of fruits, vegetables, whole grains, legumes, nuts, and seeds provides a diverse range of fibers that nourish the gut microbiome. Aim for a colorful and varied plate at each meal.

- Probiotic-Rich Foods: Incorporate probiotic-rich foods into the diet to introduce beneficial live bacteria to the gut. Yogurt, kefir, sauerkraut, kimchi, and other fermented foods contribute to microbial diversity.

- Prebiotic Foods: Include prebiotic-rich foods that serve as fuel for beneficial bacteria. Garlic, onions, leeks, bananas, asparagus, and chicory root are examples of foods that contain prebiotics.

2. Embrace a Balanced Lifestyle:

- Regular Physical Activity: Engage in regular physical activity, such as walking, jogging, or other forms of exercise. Exercise promotes gut motility and supports a diverse gut microbiome.

- Quality Sleep: Prioritize adequate and quality sleep to support overall well-being, including gut health. Establishing a consistent sleep routine and creating a conducive sleep environment contribute to restful sleep.

- Stress Management Techniques: Incorporate stress management techniques into daily life. Practices such as mindfulness meditation, deep breathing exercises, and activities that promote relaxation contribute to a healthier gut-brain axis.

3. Mindful Hydration:

- Adequate Water Intake: Ensure consistent and adequate water intake throughout the day. Hydration supports digestion, nutrient absorption, and the overall function of the digestive tract.

- Herbal Teas and Infusions: Explore herbal teas and infusions as hydrating alternatives. Some herbal teas, such as peppermint or ginger tea, may have additional benefits for digestion.

4. Limit Antibiotic Use when Possible:

- Consultation with Healthcare Professionals: When prescribed antibiotics, consult with healthcare professionals to discuss the necessity, duration, and potential impact on the gut microbiome. Follow prescribed guidelines for antibiotic use.

- Probiotic Supplementation: In cases where antibiotics are necessary, consider probiotic supplementation under the guidance of healthcare professionals. Probiotics can help restore microbial balance after antibiotic treatment.

5. Environmental Awareness:

- Reducing Chemical Exposures: Be mindful of environmental exposures to chemicals and pollutants. Choose organic produce when possible, minimize the use of harmful household chemicals, and be aware of potential exposures in the surrounding environment.

- Connection with Nature: Spend time in nature to promote overall well-being. Exposure to natural environments has been associated with positive effects on mental health and may indirectly benefit the gut through the gut-brain axis.

6. Regular Monitoring and Professional Guidance:

- Symptom Awareness: Stay attuned to gut health by monitoring symptoms such as changes in bowel habits, bloating, or abdominal discomfort. Promptly address any persistent or concerning symptoms.

- Healthcare Professional Consultation: Consult with healthcare professionals for personalized guidance on gut health. If experiencing persistent digestive issues or seeking to optimize gut wellness, healthcare professionals can offer tailored recommendations.

7. Continuous Learning and Adaptation:

- Stay Informed: Stay informed about emerging research and insights related to gut health. The field of microbiome science is dynamic, and ongoing learning allows individuals to make informed choices.

- Adaptation to Individual Needs: Recognize that individual responses to dietary and lifestyle factors can vary. Adopt an adaptable approach, making adjustments based on personal preferences, tolerances, and responses.

Sustaining long-term gut wellness is a journey of intentional choices, mindful practices, and a holistic understanding of the dynamic interplay between the gut microbiome and overall health. As we navigate this journey, it becomes clear that gut wellness is not a destination but a continuous process of nourishing, balancing, and adapting.

In embracing the principles of a plant-rich diet, balanced lifestyle, mindful hydration, and environmental awareness, we cultivate an environment where the gut microbiome thrives. We

honor the symbiotic relationship between the human host and its microbial inhabitants—a relationship that extends beyond digestion to influence immunity, metabolism, and mental well-being.

As we prioritize sustained gut wellness, let us do so with a sense of empowerment and curiosity. Let us celebrate the vibrant colors of plant-based meals, relish the joy of physical activity, and savor the tranquility of a well-nourished gut-brain axis. In this ongoing exploration, may we find not only digestive harmony but a profound connection to the innate wisdom of our bodies—a wisdom that invites us to listen, adapt, and thrive in the ever-changing landscape of long-term gut wellness.

www.ingramcontent.com/pod-product-compliance
Lightning Source LLC
Chambersburg PA
CBHW071005260726
48661CB00007B/2807